Adventures of David and Joshua

Facing the Storm

Story provided by Terence, Eardie, David and Joshua Houston

Illustrated by Laura Acosta

Revised and edited by Shyreeta Benbow

TDR Brands Publishing

Living Life with the Houston's
14019 SW Freeway
Suite 301-197
Sugar Land, TX 77478

Please visit www.livinglifewiththehoustons.com to get connected

Printed in the United States of America

ISBN 978-1-947574-15-1

Dedicated to Bernetta, Theodore, and Sarah. Thank you for teaching us about faith and fortitude. Love to our siblings, Bernetta, Ian, and Ilona.

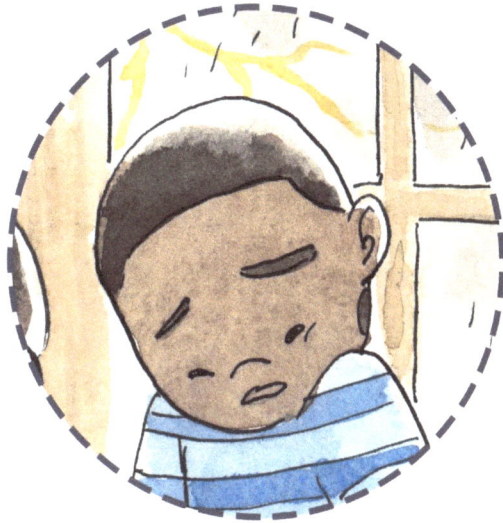

Adventures of David and Joshua

Facing the Storm

Facing the Storm

Before it began to rain, David and Joshua were outside playing. Mommy saw the dark clouds outside and went to call the boys inside.

"David and Joshua, it's time to come inside!" said Mommy.

"Do we really have to come inside now mommy?" asked Joshua.

Mommy said, "It's going to rain really hard and I don't want you guys to get wet. Do you see how dark the sky is?"

"Yes, Mommy!" both boys said as they ran inside of the house.

"Boys, slow down before you hurt yourself!" said Mommy.

As they ran inside, Mommy told the boys to go and get cleaned up for dinner.

David's job was to clean and clear off the table. Joshua's job was to place the plates, spoons, and napkins on the table for dinner.

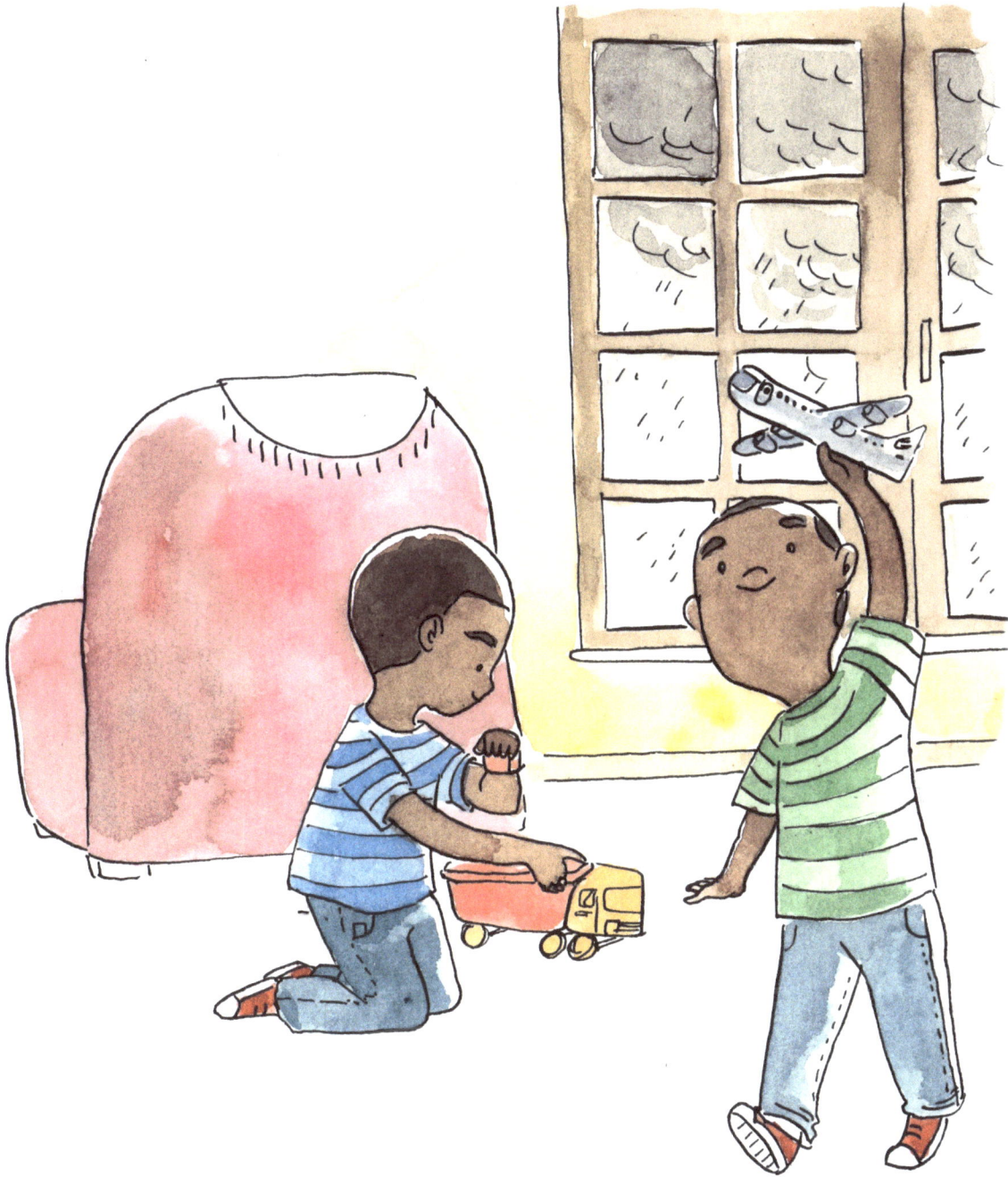

"Did you guys clear off the table and put down the plates, spoons, and napkins?" said Mommy.

"Yes!" said David and Joshua.

"Great job following directions boys!" said Mommy.

"Thank you, Mommy!" said David and then Joshua.

"We will play a game after dinner and you guys get to choose!" said Mommy.

"YAY, I love playing games! Can we play Twister?" said Joshua.

"I don't want to play Twister! Can we play Legos?" said David with his hand up.

Mommy said, "We have to all agree on one game so that it will be fair and fun for us all."

David and Joshua sat at the table, thinking.

They both screamed out, "THE MATCHING GAME!"

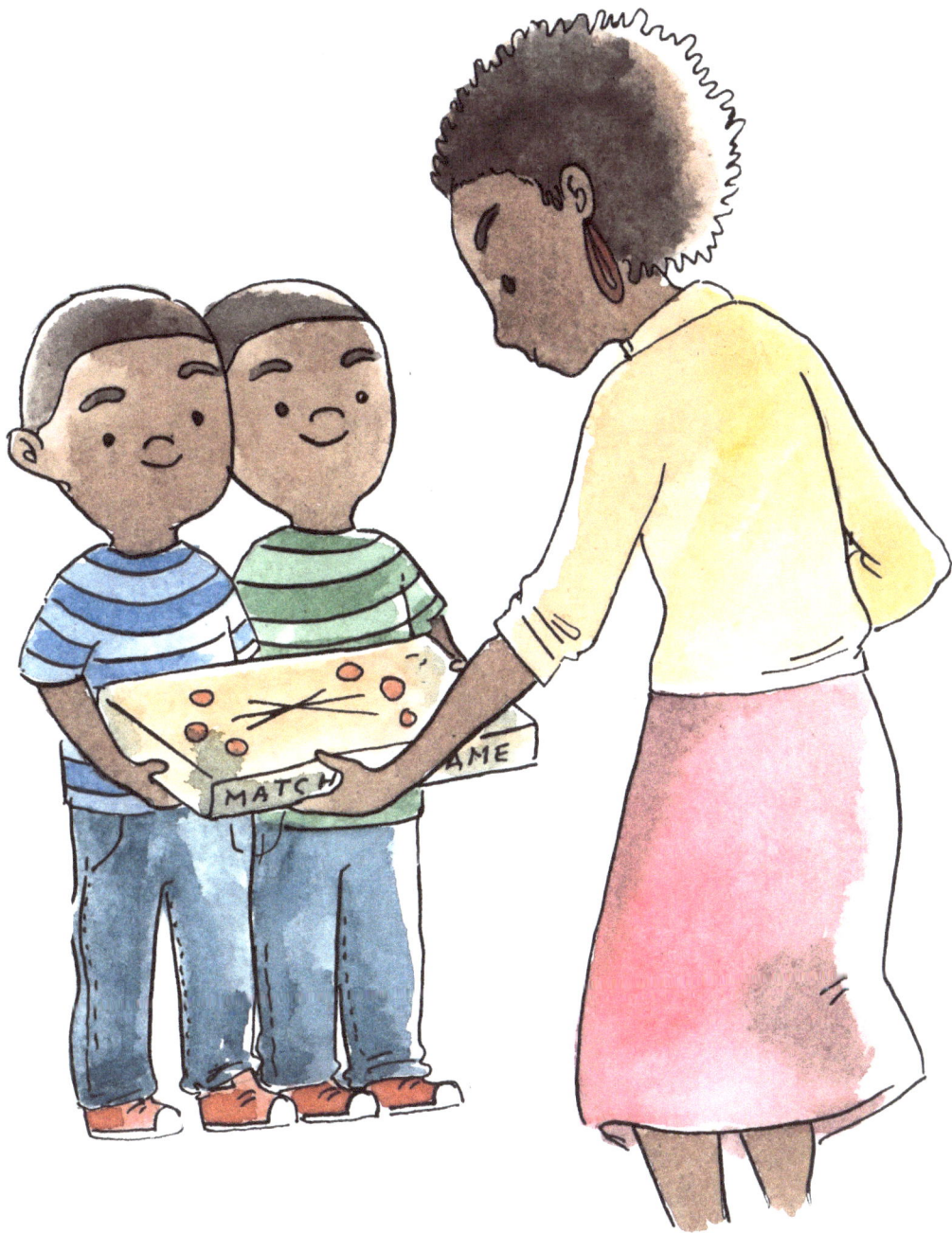

Dinner was over and the family went into the living room to play.

The kids went to the window and were really happy to see a BIG rainbow across the sky. They were amazed!

"Mommy, look, a rainbow!" said David.

"I've never seen a rainbow before Mommy!" said Joshua.

"It's beautiful, isn't it?" Mommy said.

"Yes!" the boys said slowly.

"Ok, now let's get this game started boys." said Mommy. As they sat and played the matching game, the lights in the house went off and then on again.

There was a big BOOM sound as it started to rain really hard.

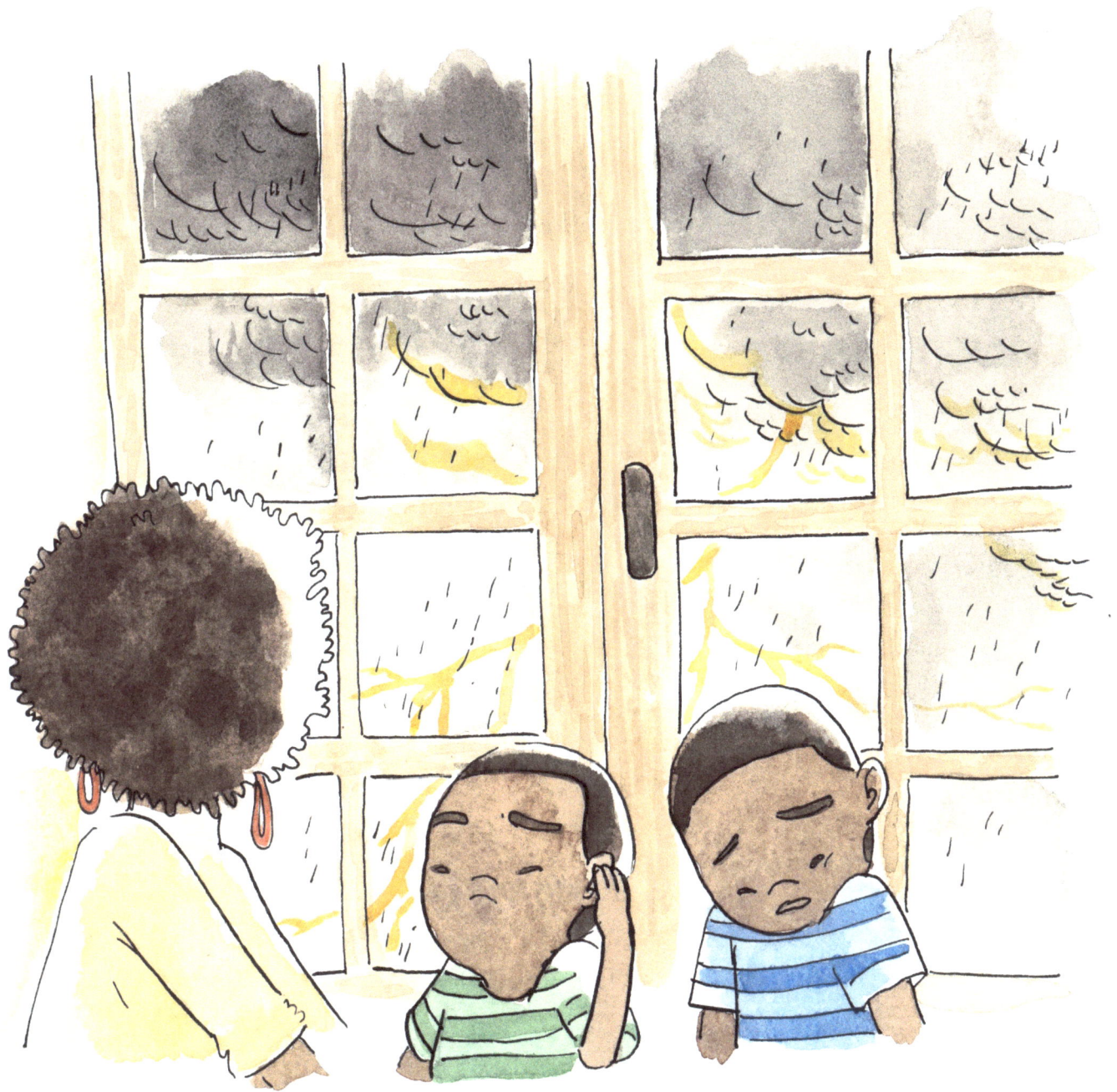

Joshua ran to his Mommy and put his head under her arm. He was really afraid.

"Mommy, I'm scared!" Joshua said as he started to shake.

"It's alright Joshua, Mommy's here. We are safely inside from the thunder and lightning." said Mommy.

"It's ok Joshua and Mommy. I am here to protect you both until Dad gets home. I will go and get the flashlight." said David.

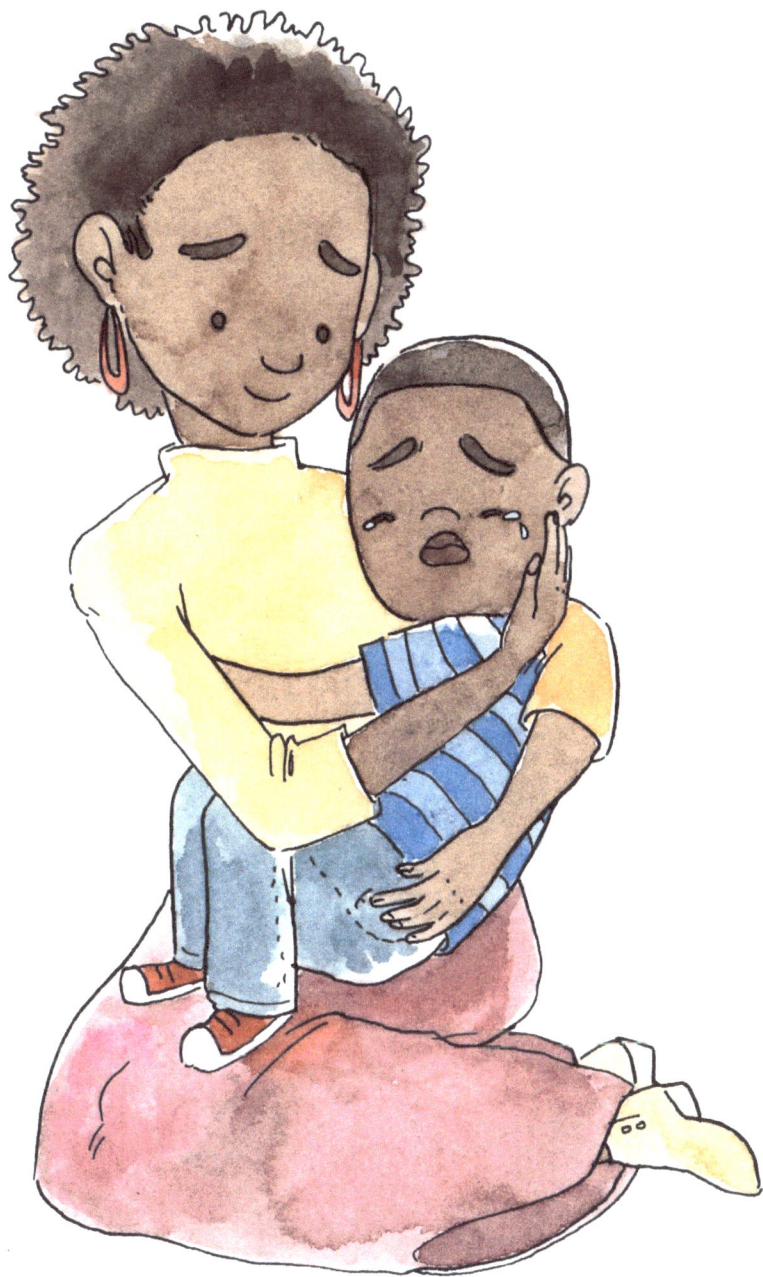

"I want my Daddy!" Joshua cried.

"Daddy will be home soon, Joshua. If it gets too bad, we will go down to the basement. You know how they taught you during the tornado drill at school? We will do it at home, too" said Mommy.

David looked out the window and just like that, the loud thunder and scary lightning was gone. There was another rainbow in the sky.

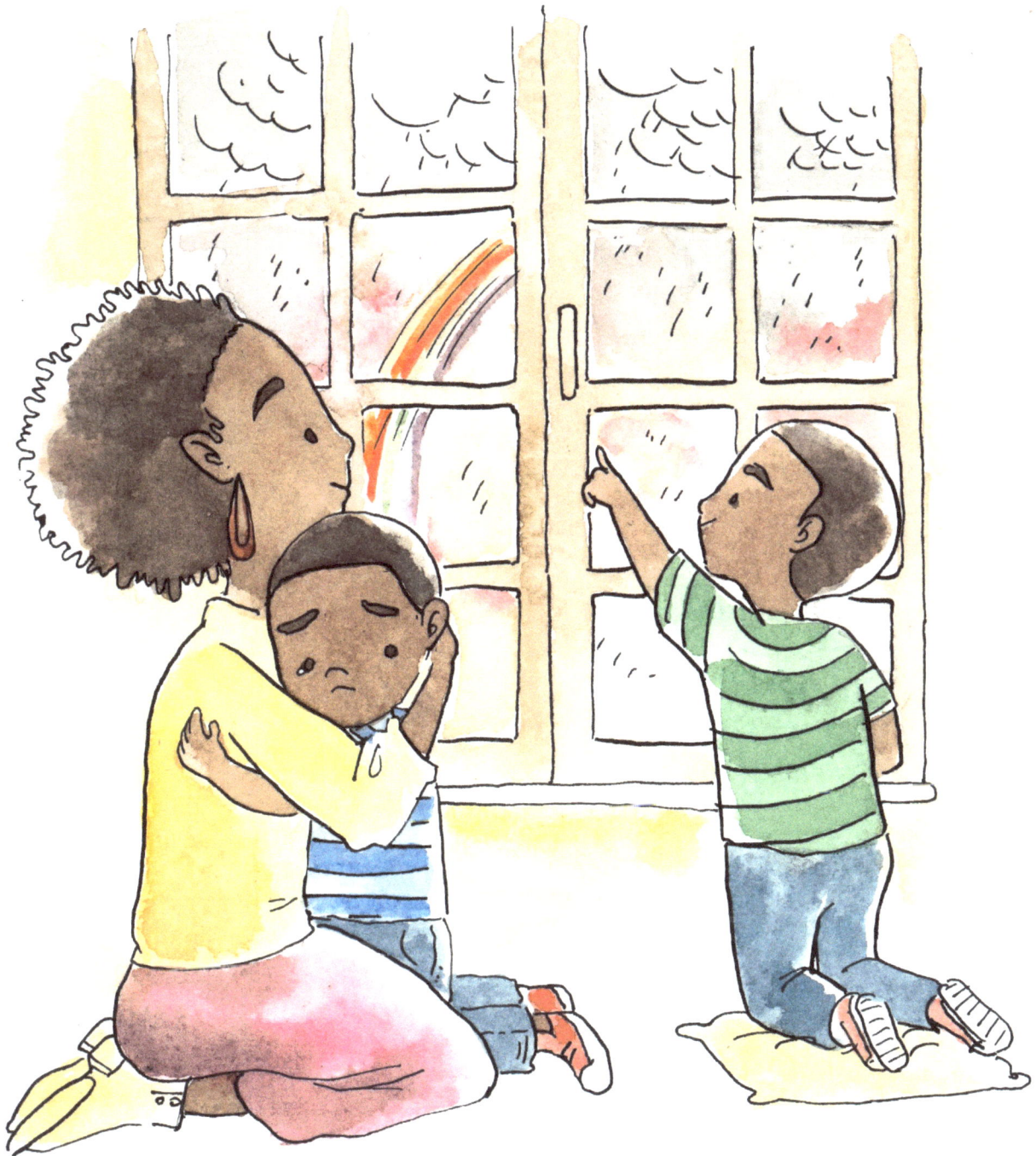

"Joshua! Mommy! LOOK! There's another BIG rainbow in the sky!" David said with excitement.

Joshua looked up, but didn't want to go to the window.

David grabbed Joshua by the hand, and said, "It's OK, Joshua. The lightning is all gone now. Come see."

Joshua wiped his face and went to look out of the window with his brother. "But it's still raining", Joshua mumbled.

"Don't focus on the storm, Joshua. Just focus on the rainbow! It's less scary that way", said David.

Mommy watched her brave boys, and smiled to herself as they encouraged each other. David's wise words encouraged Mommy, too, as she repeated them to herself. "Don't focus on the storm. Just focus on the rainbow."

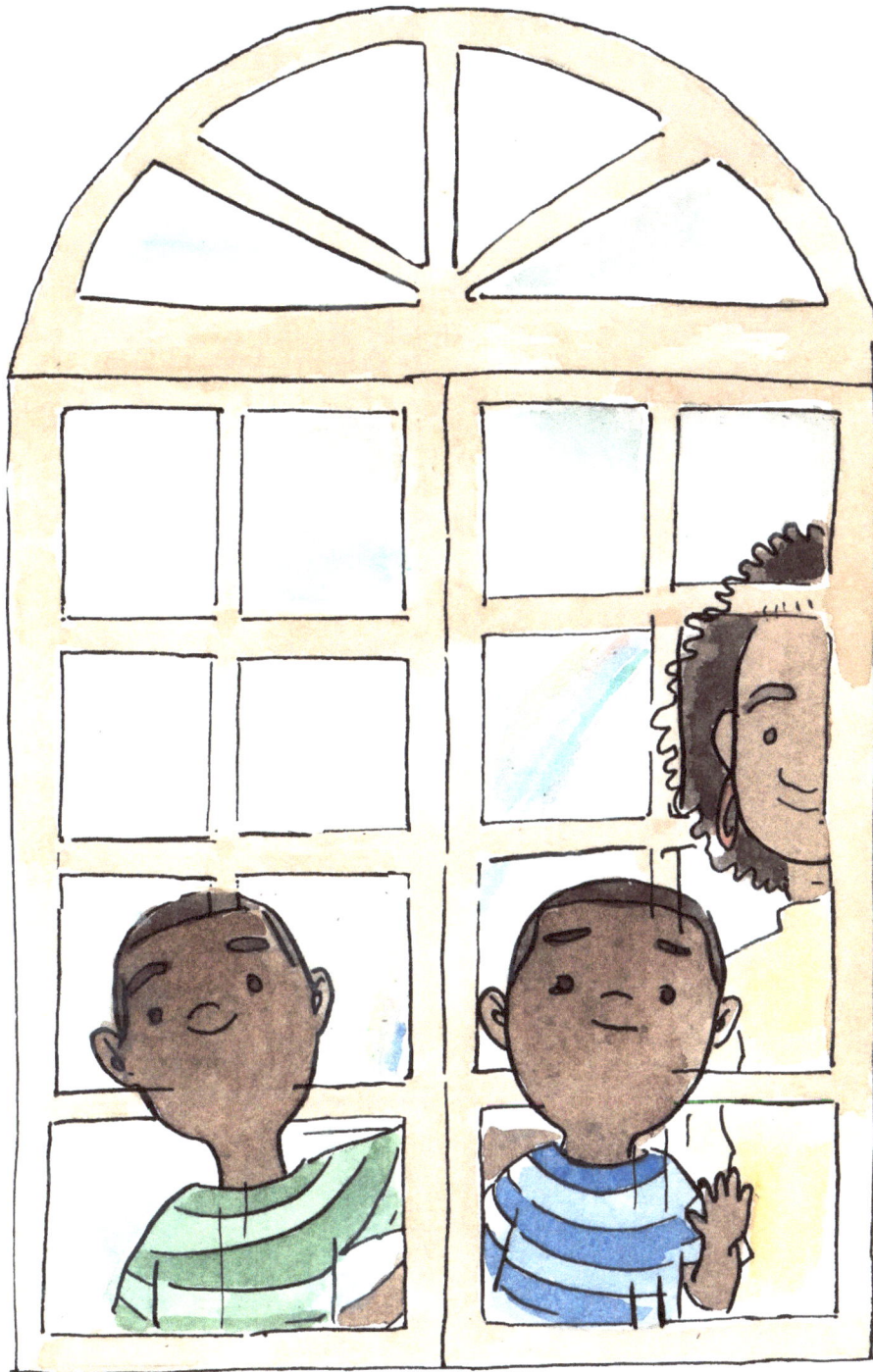

The End

"This is my command – be strong and courageous! Do not be afraid or discouraged. For the LORD your God is with you wherever you go."

Joshua 1:9 NLT

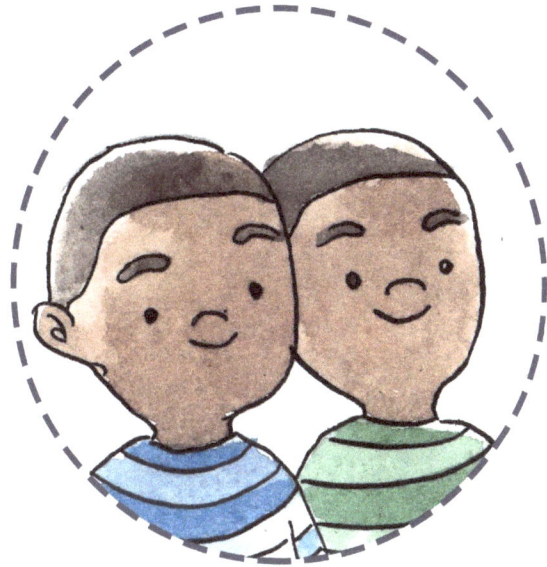

The Houston's reside in Houston Texas and are on a mission to educate, inspire, and serve their community.

Please visit www.livinglifewiththehoustons.com to join our community and let us know what you think and send your feedback, inquiries, and collaboration opportunities to
contact@livinglifewiththehoustons.com

Join our email newsletter today for a free surprise from David and Joshua!

Keep enjoying fun stories with other books from the series "Adventures of David and Joshua" and "Chronicles of Christian Grace".
To request bulk orders or book signing request, please visit our website.

www.ingramcontent.com/pod-product-compliance
Lightning Source LLC
Chambersburg PA
CBHW060856270326
41934CB00002B/157